Weight Watchers Slow Cooker

Easy Crockpot Recipes for Rapid Weight Loss

Madison Miller

Copyrights

All rights reserved © Madison Miller and The Cookbook Publisher. No part of this publication or the information in it may be quoted from or reproduced in any form by means such as printing, scanning, photocopying, or otherwise without prior written permission of the copyright holder.

Disclaimer and Terms of Use

Effort has been made to ensure that the information in this book is accurate and complete. However, the author and the publisher do not warrant the accuracy of the information, text, and graphics contained within the book due to the rapidly changing nature of science, research, known and unknown facts, and internet. The author and the publisher do not hold any responsibility for errors, omissions, or contrary interpretation of the subject matter herein. This book is presented solely for motivational and informational purposes only.

The recipes provided in this book are for informational purposes only and are not intended to provide dietary advice. A medical practitioner should be consulted before making any changes in diet. Additionally, recipe cooking times may require adjustment depending on age and quality of appliances. Readers are strongly urged to take all precautions to ensure ingredients are fully cooked in order to avoid the dangers of foodborne illnesses. The recipes and suggestions provided in this book are solely the opinion of the author. The author and publisher do not take any responsibility for any consequences that may result due to following the instructions provided in this book.

ISBN: 978-1537248523

Printed in the United States

— THE —
COOK BOOK
PUBLISHER

Avant-Propos

One of the biggest challenges we face when it comes to healthy eating is finding the time and energy to make healthy meals from scratch, using wholesome ingredients that complement our diets, rather than sabotaging them. Even a plan like Weight Watchers®, which is created specifically to achieve results without being overly complicated, can pose challenges at the end of a busy day. This book of slow cooker meals helps to eliminate this challenge. This book is full of healthy and delicious recipes that are nutritionally packed and suitable for any sensible healthy eating plan. Complete with Weight Watchers® **SmartPoint™** values, this book of creative, fix-it-and-leave-it meals will bring new life and inspiration to your healthy eating and weight loss goals.

Ler's get cooking,

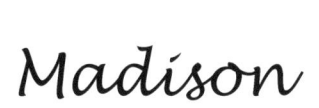

Madison

Contents

Introduction 1
   A Few Slow Cooker Tips 4
Soups and Stews 9
   Hearty Beef and Vegetable Soup 9
   Chicken Taco Soup 11
   Meatball Stroganoff Soup 13
   Kicky Asian Chicken Soup 15
   South American Beef Stew 17
   Salmon Chowder 19
   Pork and Tart Apple Stew 21
Chicken 23
   Insane Garlic Chicken 23
   Summer Chicken Provence 24
   BBQ Chicken and Purple Vegetables 25
   Parmesan Asiago Chicken with Mushrooms and
   Asparagus 27
   Peachy Mustard Chicken 29
   Chicken Tikka Masala 31
   Leek and Bok Choy Chicken 33
   Smokey Mexican Chicken 35
   Mango Chicken Salad 37
Pork 39
   Cranberry Apple Tenderloin 39
   Chinese BBQ Shredded Pork 41
   Honey Cuban Pork 43
   Pork and Quinoa Cabbage Rolls 45
   Balsamic Fig Pork Chops 47
   Mediterranean Pork Roast 49
   Jamaican Tenderloin 51
   Italian Style Spareribs 53
Beef and Lamb 55
   Saucy Garden Steaks 55
   Brisket and Cabbage Dinner 57
   Gingery Asian Sloppy Joes 59
   Mushroomy Pot Roast 61

- Tri Tip Fajitas 63
- Dark Cherry Beef Roast 65
- Curried Lamb 67
- Eggplant and Lamb 69
- Dijon Brisket 71

Vegetarian 73
- Quinoa Casserole with Mushrooms and Artichokes ... 73
- Ratatouille 75
- Colorful Vegetable Risotto 77
- Basil Angel Hair Frittata 79
- Chayote and Quinoa Stuffed Peppers 81
- Chickpea Chili 83
- Veggie Fajita Salad 85
- Vegetable Gumbo 87
- Greek Succotash 89

Conclusion 91
More Books from Madison Miller 93
Appendix – Cooking Conversion Charts 95

Introduction

If you are reading this book, then chances are you have decided to make big changes in your life, or are already in the process of making those changes. As a society, we are growing larger, not just in numbers, but also in waist circumference. Obesity rates across the United States are at an all-time high and come with significant health consequences. However, the truth is that you do not need to be considered obese to suffer the ill effects of carrying around a few too many extra pounds. Being overweight even by ten or twenty pounds can cause fatigue, depression, stress, anxiety, blood sugar irregularities, high blood pressure and stress on the supportive tissues in your body, just to name a few. While our bodies are growing larger, so it seems is our desire to regain our health and feel good about who we see physically when we look in the mirror.

Making the decision to become healthier and follow a specific dietary plan is easy; you simply decide you want to do it. It is the follow through that is often the most difficult. Take a look around in your local bookstore, online or through any source of media and you will find a selection of dietary plan options that is so vast that it is almost dizzying. There are fruit, juice, or vegetable fasts, diets that focus on only one or two foods, diets that restrict calories, diets that restrict carbs, diets that restrict sugar, diets that promote ancient eating patterns and eliminate much of the food that is available today. Choosing which plan to follow and knowing which one is best for your body is a challenge that can be frustrating, if not impossible to achieve on your own without sound advice. Many people try, searching diet after diet, for the miracle plan that will melt pounds off of their bodies as effortlessly as possible. Most of the time, the result of this is frustration and (although I hate to use the word) failure.

The reason we fail at diets is simple. They are not designed to promote lifelong healthy eating habits. You can restrict calories to lose weight, but how long will you be able to maintain that, or how long can you continue to do that without sending your metabolism into a state of havoc? You can restrict the foods you eat, but without necessary medical reasons, chances are that you will soon grow bored and resort back to your old eating patterns. This is why when you approach a professional, such as your doctor or a dietician, they will tell you that fad diets don't work and the best approach is a modification that focuses on healthy choices and portion sizes without putting unrealistic expectations on you or forcing you to count every calorie or carbohydrate that passes your lips. It is for this reason that the Weight Watchers® plan has been one of the most successful and a favorite of medical professionals for years.

Choosing a successful plan like Weight Watchers® only solves part of the problem. Another reason why so many diets is fail is that they are complicated and simply take too much time to do the meal planning, grocery shopping, preparation, etc. This is where the recipes in this book are going to make a big change in your life. With the Weight Watchers® plan, you can eat whatever you want. Each food, or recipe, is assigned a point value. All you need to do is stay within your specially assigned point range for your health and fitness goals. Eating whatever you want, whenever you want sound great. But still, making delicious, wholesome meals at home can take more time and energy than many of us have available at the end of our busy days. Whether your days are spent at the office, or running around taking care of the endless needs of children, or both, chances are dinner time comes and you are exhausted. When presented with the choice of spending time and energy in the kitchen, or maybe instead, cheating "just a little" and going for something fast, processed and out of your point budget—without the proper incentive, it becomes quite easy to choose the latter.

Within this book you will find the solution to this problem. Rather than spending too much time in the kitchen, you can spend just a few minutes earlier in the day and be rewarded with a scrumptious home cooked meal come dinner time. This book of slow cooker recipes was designed not only to provide you with low point options for healthy and delicious meals, but also make bringing these meals to your dinner table an easy reality. With little preparation and easy-to-find ingredients, you will never be able to use the excuse of not having enough time or being bored with your choices. Making healthy choices is actually the easiest and quickest choice of all, once you know how to do it and are aware of the endless options available to you, especially with the use of your slow cooker.

A Few Slow Cooker Tips

If you are a veteran slow cooker user, then you likely know all the little nuances that come with this incredible appliance. However, some of you will pick up this book and a new slow cooker at the same time. You have made a wonderful choice. You will be amazed at how easy it is to prepare food that is nutritious and pleasing to your taste buds as well as your scale. Following are just a few tips to help you get started in slow cooking.

Not all slow cookers are created equal.

Do a little research and find one that fits your needs, as well as one that has good customer reviews. Some slow cookers have a simple "LOW" and "HIGH" setting. Others will have more choices in temperature range and timing options. The recipes in this book have been designed to work with the most basic of slow cookers; however, if you plan on using your slow cooker quite often you might want to look into one with a little more variability. Also, consider size. Ask yourself questions like how big is your kitchen, will you keep it out when it is not in use or will you store it, how big is your family, how much food will you cook at once, are you looking to make extra and freeze it for later, etc. Slow cookers come in various sizes. The recipes in this book have been created for use in five to seven quart slow cookers, or larger.

Just because you throw it all in one pot, that doesn't mean it will all cook evenly.

You want as even cooking over the duration of the cooking period as possible. This means that foods that are cut, such as vegetables, should be cut according to cooking time. For example, a quicker cooking vegetable should be cut into larger pieces while slower cooking vegetables should be cut into smaller pieces. Some ingredients, such as peas or spinach, cook quickly enough that many times they can be added near the end of the cooking time to avoid them becoming too mushy or disintegrating completely during the cooking process.

Keep food safety in mind.

Cooking times given should be considered to be approximate, not set in stone. Your food might be thicker, or cut in a different way and your slow cooker might cook at a slightly different temperature than other models. Just like some ovens cook differently, so do slow cookers. For this reason, a good quality food thermometer is a good investment. As a general rule, you want meats to register at 165°F, especially for poultry. Cook beef according to temperature preferences, but use caution when handling beef that is more on the rare side.

Placement is key.

You will notice that in some of the recipes, the meat is placed on the bottom with the vegetables on top or surrounding the meat. In other recipes, the order is reversed. Sometimes a sauce is added first, sometimes it is added last. There really is a reason for the method and it is all about what the final product will be. Generally, you want meats close to the bottom so they have more exposure to the heat source, since they typically take longer to cook. There are some recipes though, that depend on the juices of the meat dripping down over the vegetables for a specific flavor or texture.

A little moisture is good thing.

You do not need to drench each dish with cups of liquid, but it is always a good idea to add at least half a cup of liquid to the slow cooker. This will help prevent dryness or burning.

Not all foods make for a good slow cooker meal.

Fish and seafood can be cooked in a slow cooker, but require a much, much lower cooking time. Where beef or chicken might take four to eight hours, shrimp would take an hour or less. Many people find that the convenience of the slow cooker lies in the fill-it-and-leave-it-for-hours method. This doesn't really apply for fish and seafood. Don't get me wrong – you can create delicious seafood dishes in a slow cooker, it just takes a different approach. Another type of ingredient that doesn't do well in slow cookers is dairy. You can get away with a little dairy, but adding a significant quantity of dairy and leaving it in the slow cooker for hours will often result in a broken, curdled mess. When using dairy in your dishes, try adding it towards the end of cooking time for better results.

Make it even easier on yourself.

If you are a meal planner, prepping the ingredients early will make slow cooker cooking even easier. Cut vegetables and even season them ahead of time and all you need to do is toss and go.

Try searing the meat first.

Searing meats in a skillet with a little bit of olive oil before adding them to the slow cooker will help keep juices in and result in a more flavorful and tender piece of meat.

Enjoy and experiment.

Keep these tips in mind and try out some of your own ideas. You will have years of memorable meals with your slow cooker.

Soups and Stews

Hearty Beef and Vegetable Soup

Cook Time: 6 hours
Serves: 6
SmartPoint™: 6

Ingredients:
1 pound beef steak, cubed
1 tablespoon olive oil
½ teaspoon salt
1 teaspoon coarsely ground black pepper
1 teaspoon garlic powder
2 cups sweet potatoes, peeled and cubed
2 cups tomatoes, chopped
2 cups carrots, sliced
½ cup onion, diced
1 cup edamame, shelled
1 cup fresh green beans, trimmed
3 cloves garlic, crushed and minced
1 sprig fresh rosemary
2 cups beef stock
2 cups tomato juice

Directions:
1. Place the olive oil in a skillet over medium-high heat.
2. Season the beef steak with salt, black pepper, and garlic powder.
3. Add the beef to the skillet and brown for 3-4 minutes. Remove from the heat and transfer the steak cubes into a slow cooker.

4. On top of the meat, add the sweet potatoes, tomatoes, carrots, onion, edamame, green beans, garlic, and rosemary.
5. Pour in the beef stock and tomato juice. If more broth is desired, add additional water until the desired amount is reached.
6. Cover the slow cooker and cook on HIGH for 6 hours.

Nutritional Information:
Calories 264, Total Fat 6 g, Saturated Fat 1 g, Total Carbohydrate 27 g, Dietary Fiber 4 g, Sugars 5 g, Protein 24 g

Chicken Taco Soup

Cook Time: 6 hours
Serves: 6
SmartPoint™: 5

Ingredients:
1 pound ground chicken
½ teaspoon salt
1 teaspoon black pepper
1 teaspoon cumin
1 teaspoon chili powder
1 tablespoon lime juice
1 cup red onion, diced
1 cup green bell pepper, diced
1 cup fresh or jarred spicy tomato salsa
4 cups tomato juice
½ cup scallions, sliced
½ cup fresh tomato, diced
Shredded cheese (optional)
Avocado, cubed (optional)

Directions:
1. Place the ground chicken in a slow cooker and season it with the salt, black pepper, cumin, chili powder, and lime juice. Toss to mix the seasoning into the meat.
2. Add the onion, green bell pepper, and tomato salsa. Stir to combine.
3. Top with the tomato juice.
4. Cover the slow cooker and cook on LOW for 6 hours.
5. Serve garnished with scallions, tomatoes, and optional cheese and avocado, if desired.

Nutritional Information:
Calories 191, Total Fat 8 g, Saturated Fat 2 g, Total Carbohydrate 14 g, Dietary Fiber 2 g, Sugars 5 g, Protein 16 g

Meatball Stroganoff Soup

Cook Time: 6 ½ hours
Serves: 8
SmartPoint™: 5

Ingredients:
½ pound ground chicken
½ pound ground turkey
1 egg, lightly beaten
2 tablespoons fresh chives
1 teaspoon salt
1 teaspoon black pepper
1 tablespoon olive oil
3 cups fresh assorted mushrooms, sliced thick
1 cup onion, sliced thin
4 cups beef broth
2 tablespoons tomato paste
½ cup low fat sour cream
½ cup low fat cream cheese
¼ cup Parmesan cheese
¼ cup fresh parsley, chopped

Directions:
1. In a bowl, combine the ground chicken and ground turkey along with the egg, chives, salt, and black pepper. Mix well.
2. Form the mixture into meatballs measuring no more than one inch in diameter.
3. Heat the olive oil in a skillet over medium-high heat.
4. Add the meatballs to the skillet and cook, turning frequently, until evenly browned on all sides.

5. Remove the meatballs from the skillet and transfer to a slow cooker.
6. Top the meatballs with the mushrooms and onion.
7. Combine the beef broth and tomato paste. Mix well and pour into the slow cooker.
8. Cover and cook on LOW for six hours.
9. Remove the cover and stir in the sour cream, cream cheese, Parmesan cheese and parsley. Replace the cover and continue cooking for an additional 30 minutes before serving.

Nutritional Information:
Calories 203, Total Fat 11 g, Saturated Fat 3 g, Total Carbohydrate 6 g, Dietary Fiber 1 g, Sugars 2 g, Protein 20 g

Kicky Asian Chicken Soup

Cook Time: 6 hours
Serves: 6
SmartPoint™: 5

Ingredients:
1 pound boneless, skinless chicken breast, cubed
1 teaspoon black pepper
½ teaspoon coriander
1 teaspoon crushed red pepper
1 cup red bell pepper, sliced
1 cup onion, sliced
1 cup carrot, thinly sliced
4 cups chicken or vegetable stock
1 tablespoon ponzu or soy sauce
1 tablespoon freshly grated ginger
1 tablespoon garlic chili paste
1 ½ cup frozen edamame, shelled
2 cups Napa cabbage, shredded

Directions:
1. Place the chicken breast in a slow cooker and season it with black pepper, coriander, and crushed red pepper. Toss to mix.
2. Add the red bell pepper, onion, and carrot.
3. In a bowl, combine the chicken or vegetable stock, ponzu or soy sauce, ginger and garlic chili paste. Mix well and pour into the slow cooker.
4. Cover and cook on LOW for 5 ½ hours.
5. Remove the cover and add the edamame and Napa cabbage.

6. Replace the cover and cook an additional 30-40 minutes, or until the newly added vegetables are tender.

Nutritional Information:
Calories 230, Total Fat 5 g, Saturated Fat 1 g, Total Carbohydrate 17 g, Dietary Fiber 2 g, Sugars 5 g, Protein 27 g

South American Beef Stew

Cook Time: 5 hours
Serves: 6
SmartPoint™: 7

Ingredients:
1 ½ pounds beef steak or stew meat, cubed
1 teaspoon salt
1 teaspoon black pepper
½ teaspoon coriander
½ teaspoon nutmeg
½ teaspoon cayenne powder
2 cups carrots, sliced
2 cups ripe tomatoes, chopped
2 cups sweet potato, cubed
1 cup pumpkin, cubed
1 cup green bell pepper, chopped
1 cup onion, chopped
2 cloves garlic, crushed and minced
4 cups beef stock
2 cups cabbage, sliced thin

Directions:
1. Place the beef in a slow cooker and season with the salt, black pepper, coriander, nutmeg, and cayenne powder. Mix well.
2. Add the carrots, tomatoes, sweet potatoes, pumpkin, green bell pepper, onion, and garlic.
3. Cover the meat and vegetables with the beef stock and place the cover on the slow cooker.
4. Cook on HIGH for 4 hours.

5. Remove the cover and add the cabbage. Replace the cover and cook an additional 30 minutes before serving.

Nutritional Information:
Calories 277, Total Fat 5 g, Saturated Fat 1 g, Total Carbohydrate 26 g, Dietary Fiber 5 g, Sugars 3 g, Protein 31 g

Salmon Chowder

Cook Time: 4 hours
Serves: 6
SmartPoint™: 5

Ingredients:
1 pound salmon steak, cubed
1 teaspoon salt
1 teaspoon black pepper
1 teaspoon onion powder
1 teaspoon smoked paprika
2 cups potatoes, cubed
½ cup onion, chopped
2 cups broccoli florets
1 cup red bell pepper, chopped
2 cups vegetable or chicken stock
2 cups low fat milk
¼ cup instant mashed potatoes (optional, for thickening)

Directions:
1. Season the salmon steak with salt, black pepper, onion powder, and paprika. Place the salmon in a slow cooker.
2. Next, add the potatoes, onion, broccoli florets, and red bell pepper.
3. Pour in the vegetable stock, cover, and cook on HIGH for 3 ½ hours.
4. Remove the cover and stir in the milk and instant mashed potatoes, if using. Return the cover and cook for an additional 30 minutes.

Nutritional Information:
Calories 196, Total Fat 3 g, Saturated Fat 1 g, Total Carbohydrate 16 g, Dietary Fiber 2 g, Sugars 6 g, Protein 24 g

Pork and Tart Apple Stew

Cook Time: 8 hours
Serves: 8
SmartPoint™: 6

Ingredients:
1 ½ pounds pork tenderloin, cubed
1 teaspoon salt
1 teaspoon black pepper
½ teaspoon cinnamon
1 teaspoon ground caraway seed
2 cups sweet potatoes, cubed
1 cup carrots, sliced
1 cup onion, sliced
1 ½ cups Granny Smith apple, coarsely chopped
1 cup chicken or vegetable stock
2 cups apple cider or apple juice

Directions:
1. Season the pork tenderloin cubes with salt, black pepper, cinnamon, and caraway. Toss to mix and place in a slow cooker.
2. Cover the meat with sweet potatoes, carrots, onion, and apples.
3. Combine the chicken stock and apple cider or juice, and then pour it over the contents of the slow cooker.
4. Cover and cook on LOW for 8 hours.

Nutritional Information:
Calories 270, Total Fat 7 g, Saturated Fat 1 g, Total Carbohydrate 22 g, Dietary Fiber 2 g, Sugars 3 g, Protein 26 g

Chicken

Insane Garlic Chicken

Cook Time: 6 hours
Serves: 4
SmartPoint™: 3

Ingredients:
1 pound boneless, skinless chicken breast
1 tablespoon lemon juice
¼ cup dry white wine
1 teaspoon salt
1 teaspoon black pepper
10 whole garlic cloves
½ cup onion, sliced
½ cup green bell pepper, sliced
¼ cup fresh basil, chopped

Directions:
1. Place the chicken breast in a slow cooker.
2. In a bowl, combine the lemon juice, dry white wine, salt, black pepper, and garlic cloves. Mix well.
3. Pour the mixture over the chicken, turning the chicken breast to evenly distribute the garlic.
4. Add the onion and green bell pepper.
5. Cover and cook on LOW for 6 hours.
6. Stir in the fresh basil 10 minutes before serving.

Nutritional Information:
Calories 154, Total Fat 3 g, Saturated Fat 1 g, Total Carbohydrate 1 g, Dietary Fiber 0 g, Sugars 0 g, Protein 25 g

Summer Chicken Provence

Cook Time: 6 hours
Serves: 4
SmartPoint™: 4

Ingredients:
1 pound skinless, bone in chicken pieces
½ teaspoon salt
1 teaspoon white pepper
¼ cup dry white wine
1 cup chicken stock
4 cloves garlic
2 tablespoons shallots, diced
1 tablespoons herbs de Provence
2 cups zucchini, sliced
2 cups summer squash, sliced
1 cup Roma tomatoes, sliced

Directions:
1. Season the chicken with salt and white pepper and then place it in a slow cooker.
2. Sprinkle the chicken with the dry white wine and pour in the chicken stock.
3. Add the garlic, shallots, herbs de Provence, zucchini, summer squash, and tomatoes.
4. Cover and cook on LOW for 6 hours.

Nutritional Information:
Calories 201, Total Fat 4 g, Saturated Fat 1 g, Total Carbohydrate 9 g, Dietary Fiber 2 g, Sugars 3 g, Protein 28 g

BBQ Chicken and Purple Vegetables

Cook Time: 8 hours
Serves: 6
SmartPoint™: 5

Ingredients:
1 pound skinless, bone-in chicken pieces
1 tablespoon tomato paste
1 tablespoon Dijon mustard
1 cup chicken stock
¼ cup apple cider vinegar
2 tablespoons honey
1 tablespoon crushed red pepper flakes
2 cloves garlic, crushed and minced
2 cups purple carrots, sliced
2 cups purple potato, cubed
½ teaspoon salt
1 teaspoon coarsely ground black pepper

Directions:
1. Place the chicken pieces in a slow cooker.
2. In a bowl, combine the tomato paste, Dijon mustard, chicken stock, apple cider vinegar, honey, crushed red pepper flakes, and garlic. Mix well.
3. Pour the sauce over the chicken, turning the chicken to coat evenly.
4. Add the purple carrots and purple potatoes on top of the chicken.
5. Season with salt and black pepper.
6. Cover and cook on LOW for 8 hours.

Nutritional Information:
Calories 183, Total Fat 2 g, Saturated Fat 1 g, Total Carbohydrate 19 g, Dietary Fiber 2 g, Sugars 9 g, Protein 19 g

Parmesan Asiago Chicken with Mushrooms and Asparagus

Cook Time: 4 hours
Serves: 6
SmartPoint™: 5

Ingredients:
1 ½ pounds boneless, skinless chicken breasts
½ teaspoon salt
1 teaspoon black pepper
½ teaspoon garlic powder
1 cup chicken stock
½ cup fat free mayonnaise
½ cup low fat sour cream
¼ cup freshly grated Parmesan cheese
¼ cup fresh Asiago cheese
2 cups cremini mushrooms, sliced
12 thin asparagus spears, trimmed
1 tablespoon lemon juice
1 tablespoon fresh chives

Directions:
1. Season the chicken with salt, black pepper, and garlic powder.
2. Place the chicken in a slow cooker. Pour the chicken stock over the chicken, cover, and cook on HIGH for 2 hours.
3. In a bowl, combine the fat free mayonnaise, low fat sour cream, Parmesan cheese and Asiago cheese.
4. Remove the lid from the slow cooker and brush the cheese mixture over both sides of the chicken breast.

5. Add the mushrooms and asparagus spears to the slow cooker.
6. Replace the cover and continue cooking on HIGH for an additional 2 hours.
7. Garnish with lemon juice and chives before serving

Nutritional Information:
Calories 247.0, Total Fat 9.4 g, Saturated Fat 2.7 g, Total Carbohydrate 7.3 g, Dietary Fiber 1.0 g, Sugars 3.1 g, Protein 31.8 g

Peachy Mustard Chicken

Cook Time: 6 hours
Serves: 6
SmartPoint™: 8

Ingredients:
1 ½ pounds boneless, skinless chicken breasts
1 cup peach nectar
½ cup Dijon mustard
1 teaspoon freshly grated ginger
¼ teaspoon cayenne powder
¼ teaspoon turmeric
¼ teaspoon cardamom
1 cup green bell pepper, sliced
1 cup onion, sliced
4 cups cooked brown rice

Directions:
1. Place the chicken in a slow cooker.
2. In a bowl, combine the peach nectar, Dijon mustard, fresh ginger, cayenne powder, turmeric, and cardamom. Mix well.
3. Pour the sauce over the chicken, turning the chicken to ensure even coverage on both sides.
4. Top with the green bell pepper and onion.
5. Cover and cook on LOW for 6 hours.
6. Heat the rice in a microwave long enough to warm through.
7. Serve the chicken and sauce over warmed brown rice.

Nutritional Information:
Calories 330, Total Fat 4 g, Saturated Fat 1 g, Total Carbohydrate 39 g, Dietary Fiber 3 g, Sugars 6 g, Protein 29 g

Chicken Tikka Masala

Cook Time: 8 hours
Serves: 6
SmartPoint™: 7

Ingredients:
2 pounds boneless, skinless chicken thighs
½ teaspoon salt
1 teaspoon white pepper
2 cups crushed tomatoes, with liquid
1 cup yellow onion, diced
1 cup carrot, diced
1 cup yellow bell pepper, sliced
4 cloves garlic, crushed and minced
3 tablespoons tomato paste
1 tablespoon garam masala
½ cup coconut milk
3 cups cooked long grain brown rice
1 lime, cut into wedges
¼ cup fresh cilantro, chopped
¼ cup scallions, sliced

Directions:
1. Season the chicken with salt and white pepper and place it in the slow cooker.
2. In a bowl, combine the crushed tomatoes, yellow onion, carrot, yellow bell pepper, garlic, tomato paste, and garam masala. Mix well.
3. Pour the mixture over the chicken and turn the chicken to ensure all of the chicken is well covered.
4. Cover the slow cooker and cook on LOW for 8 hours.

5. Remove the cover and stir in the coconut milk.
6. Serve over cooked rice, garnished with lime, cilantro, and scallions, if desired.

Nutritional Information:
Calories 329, Total Fat 5 g, Saturated Fat 1 g, Total Carbohydrate 30 g, Dietary Fiber 3 g, Sugars 2 g, Protein 37 g

Leek and Bok Choy Chicken

Cook Time: 8 hours
Serves: 6
SmartPoint™: 7

Ingredients:
2 pounds boneless, skinless chicken thighs
½ teaspoon salt
1 teaspoon coarsely ground black pepper
½ teaspoon coriander
4 cloves garlic, crushed and minced
1 cup leek, white parts only, cleaned and sliced
1 cup carrots, thinly sliced on the diagonal
½ cup apple cider vinegar
½ cup soy sauce
1 tablespoon brown sugar
1 cup shiitake mushrooms, sliced
2 cups Bok choy, sliced
3 cups cooked rice for serving

Directions:
1. Season the chicken with salt, black pepper, and coriander, and place it in the slow cooker.
2. Top the chicken with the garlic, leek, and carrots.
3. In a bowl, combine the apple cider vinegar, soy sauce, and brown sugar. Mix well and pour over the chicken and vegetables.
4. Cover and cook on LOW for 8 hours.
5. Fifteen minutes before serving, remove the cover and add the Bok choy and shiitake mushrooms.
6. Serve over cooked rice.

Nutritional Information:
Calories 321, Total Fat 5 g, Saturated Fat 1 g, Total Carbohydrate 28 g, Dietary Fiber 2 g, Sugars 2 g, Protein 38 g

Smokey Mexican Chicken

Cook Time: 6 hours
Serves: 4
SmartPoint™: 3

Ingredients:
1 pound boneless, skinless chicken breast, cut into strips
½ teaspoon salt
1 teaspoon black pepper
½ teaspoon smoked paprika
½ teaspoon onion powder
1 cup chicken stock
1 ½ cups tomatillos, quartered
¼ cup dried morita peppers
1 dried pasilla pepper
1 tablespoon lime juice
1 cup Poblano pepper, sliced
1 cup onion, sliced
Avocado, diced, for garnish (optional)
Tortillas for serving (optional)

Directions:
1. Season the chicken with salt, black pepper, smoked paprika, and onion powder. Place the seasoned chicken in the slow cooker.
2. In a blender, combine the chicken stock, tomatillos, morita and pasilla peppers, and lime juice. Blend until combined, and pour over the chicken.
3. Add the Poblano pepper and onion.
4. Cover and cook on LOW for 6 hours.
5. Serve in tortillas, garnished with avocado, if desired.

Nutritional Information:

Calories 190, Total Fat 4 g, Saturated Fat 1 g, Total Carbohydrate 8 g, Dietary Fiber 1 g, Sugars 2 g, Protein 30 g

Mango Chicken Salad

Cook Time: 8 hours
Serves: 6
SmartPoint™: 7

Ingredients:
1 cup yellow onion, sliced
1 cup mango, chopped
1 ½ pounds boneless, skinless chicken thighs
½ teaspoon salt
1 teaspoon black pepper
1 teaspoon ancho chili powder
½ teaspoon cumin
½ teaspoon cinnamon
1 tablespoon freshly grated ginger
4 cloves garlic, crushed and minced
1 cup roasted tomatoes, chopped with liquid
2 cups chicken stock
½ cup mango nectar
4 cups fresh, mixed salad greens
1 cup red bell pepper, diced
½ cup avocado, cubed
1 cup fresh pineapple, chunked
¼ cup scallions, sliced

Directions:
1. Season the chicken with salt, black pepper, ancho chili powder, cumin, and cinnamon. Place the chicken in the slow cooker.
2. Combine the ginger, garlic, roasted tomatoes, chicken stock, and mango nectar. Mix well and pour over the chicken.

3. Cover the slow cooker and cook on LOW for 8 hours.
4. Fifteen minutes before serving, remove the cover and shred the chicken.
5. Arrange the salad greens on serving plates and top with the chicken, adding the sauce as desired for a dressing.
6. Garnish the salads with red bell pepper, avocado, pineapple, and scallions before serving.

Nutritional Information:
Calories 258, Total Fat 6 g, Saturated Fat 1 g, Total Carbohydrate 20 g, Dietary Fiber 3 g, Sugars 12 g, Protein 29 g

Pork

Cranberry Apple Tenderloin

Cook Time: 8 hours
Serves: 8
SmartPoint™: 9

Ingredients:
2 pounds pork tenderloin
1 teaspoon salt
1 teaspoon black pepper
1 tablespoon olive oil
2 cups whole cranberries
1 cup apple, chopped
1 cup onion, sliced
3 cloves garlic, crushed and minced
2 cups chicken stock
½ cup apple juice
1 tablespoon fresh thyme
1 sprig fresh rosemary
4 cups cooked polenta, for serving
¼ cup walnuts, chopped (optional)

Directions:
1. Season the tenderloin with salt and black pepper.
2. Heat the olive oil in a large skillet over medium high.
3. Place the tenderloin in the skillet and cook, turning frequently, until it is evenly browned on all sides.
4. Remove the tenderloin from the skillet and place it in the slow cooker.
5. Arrange the cranberries, apples, and onion around the tenderloin.

6. Combine the garlic, chicken stock, and apple juice. Mix well and pour over the tenderloin.
7. Season with fresh thyme and rosemary.
8. Cover and cook on LOW for 8 hours.
9. Remove the tenderloin from the slow cooker and let it rest for 5 minutes before slicing.
10. Serve on polenta, drizzled with sauce from the slow cooker.
11. Garnish with walnuts before serving, if desired.

Nutritional Information:
Calories 370, Total Fat 12 g, Saturated Fat 2 g, Total Carbohydrate 24 g, Dietary Fiber 3 g, Sugars 3 g, Protein 37 g

Chinese BBQ Shredded Pork

Cook Time: 8 hours
Serves: 6
SmartPoint™: 5

Ingredients:
1 ½ pounds boneless pork roast
½ teaspoon salt
1 teaspoon black pepper
½ teaspoon cinnamon
2 teaspoons five spice powder
1 tablespoon crushed red pepper flakes
¼ cup soy sauce
1 cup chicken stock
2 teaspoons sesame oil
¼ cup sugar free ketchup
2 tablespoons honey
1 tablespoon freshly grated ginger
4 cloves garlic, crushed and minced
1 cup onion, sliced
1 cup red bell pepper, sliced
2 cups broccoli florets
2 cups green beans, trimmed

Directions:
1. Season the pork roast with the salt, black pepper, cinnamon, five spice powder, and crushed red pepper flakes. Set aside.
2. In a bowl, combine the soy sauce, chicken stock, sesame oil, ketchup, honey, ginger, and garlic. Whisk together until well blended and then pour half of the liquid into the slow cooker.

3. Place the roast in the slow cooker and pour the remaining sauce over the roast.
4. Arrange the onion, red bell pepper, broccoli florets, and green beans around and over the pork roast.
5. Cover the slow cooker and cook on LOW for 8 hours.
6. Remove the roast and let it rest 5 to 10 minutes. Shred before serving.

Nutritional information:
Calories 290, Total Fat 11g, Saturated Fat 2 g, Total Carbohydrate 13 g, Dietary Fiber 2 g, Sugars 5 g, Protein 36 g

Honey Cuban Pork

Cook Time: 6 hours
Serves: 8
SmartPoint™: 6

Ingredients:
2 pounds boneless pork chops
½ teaspoon salt
1 teaspoon black pepper
1 teaspoon oregano
1 teaspoon cumin
4 cloves garlic
¼ cup currants
1 tablespoon honey
¼ cup tomato paste
1 cup chicken stock
1 cup onion, chopped
2 cups green bell pepper
2 cups tomato, chopped
10 green olives, halved
2 ears of corn, quartered
¼ cup fresh cilantro, chopped
Rice for serving, optional

Directions:
1. Season the pork with salt, black pepper, oregano, and cumin. Place the pork evenly in the bottom of a slow cooker.
2. In a blender, combine the garlic, currants, honey, tomato paste, and chicken stock. Pulse until a sauce is formed.
3. Pour the sauce evenly over the pork in the slow cooker.

4. Add the bell pepper, tomatoes, olives, and corn to the slow cooker.
5. Cover and cook on LOW for 6 hours.
6. Garnish with cilantro and serve with cooked rice, if desired.

Nutritional Information:
Calories 275, Total Fat 10 g, Saturated Fat 3 g, Total Carbohydrate 17 g, Dietary Fiber 2 g, Sugars 7 g, Protein 26 g

Pork and Quinoa Cabbage Rolls

Cook Time: 4 hours
Serves: 6
SmartPoint™: 9

Ingredients:
1 large head green cabbage, cored
1 tablespoon olive oil
1 pound ground pork
2 cloves garlic, crushed and minced
½ teaspoon salt
1 teaspoon black pepper
1 teaspoon nutmeg
1 cup quinoa, cooked
½ cup firm goat cheese, crumbled
½ cup raisins, chopped
¼ cup fresh parsley, chopped
2 cups roasted tomatoes, with liquid, chopped
½ cup apple cider
1 tablespoon apple cider vinegar

Directions:
1. Place the cabbage leaves in a steamer basket and steam until tender, approximately 5 minutes. Remove, and set them aside.
2. Warm the olive oil in a skillet over medium heat.
3. Add the pork, and then season with the garlic, salt, black pepper, and nutmeg. Cook just until browned. Remove from the heat, let it cool slightly, and transfer it to a bowl.
4. To the pork mixture add the quinoa, goat cheese, raisins, and parsley. Toss to mix.

5. Lay out the cabbage leaves and spoon a generous portion of the pork mixture into the center of each leaf.
6. Roll the leaf, tucking in the sides, and place them seam side down in the slow cooker.
7. In a blender, combine the tomatoes, apple cider, and apple cider vinegar.
8. Pour the sauce over the cabbage.
9. Cover the slow cooker and cook on HIGH for 4 hours.

Nutritional Information:
Calories 320, Total Fat 19 g, Saturated Fat 5 g, Total Carbohydrate 20 g, Dietary Fiber 4 g, Sugars 4 g, Protein 24 g

Balsamic Fig Pork Chops

Cook Time: 4 ½ hours
Serves: 6
SmartPoint™: 5

Ingredients:
1 ½ pounds boneless pork chops
½ teaspoon salt
1 teaspoon black pepper
1 tablespoon olive oil
1 cup onion, sliced thick
1 cup fresh figs, quartered
¼ cup shallots
2 teaspoons fresh sage
½ cup balsamic vinegar
½ cup chicken stock
6 cups mixed dark salad greens, for serving
½ cup fresh parsley, chopped for garnish

Directions:
1. Season the pork chops with salt and black pepper. Arrange them in the slow cooker.
2. Heat the olive oil in a large skillet over medium heat.
3. Add the onion and fig. Sauté for approximately 3 minutes before adding the shallots and sage. Cook an additional 1-2 minutes.
4. Add the balsamic vinegar to the skillet and cook for several minutes until reduced, using a wooden spatula to loosen and remove any brown bits from the bottom of the pan.

5. Once the vinegar has reduced, add the chicken stock and bring it to a low boil. Remove the pan from the heat, allow it to cool slightly, and transfer the contents to the slow cooker.
6. Cover the slow cooker and cook HIGH for 4 hours.
7. Serve the pork and sauce with the mixed greens and garnish with fresh parsley before serving.

Nutritional Information:
Calories 240, Total Fat 11 g, Saturated Fat 2 g, Total Carbohydrate 11 g, Dietary Fiber 1 g, Sugars 3 g, Protein 29 g

Mediterranean Pork Roast

Cook Time: 8 hours
Serves: 8
SmartPoint™: 6

Ingredients:
2 pounds pork tenderloin roast
1 teaspoon salt
1 teaspoon black pepper
1 teaspoon thyme
½ cup sundried tomatoes, chopped
½ cup Kalamata olives, chopped
1 cup artichoke hearts, quartered
1 cup onion, sliced
4 cloves garlic, crushed and minced
1 tablespoon lemon juice
1 cup chicken stock

Directions:
1. Season the pork roast with salt, black pepper, and thyme.
2. Place the roast in the center of a slow cooker.
3. Add the sundried tomatoes, Kalamata olives, artichoke hearts, and onion. Make sure the roast is as surrounded and covered as possible with the additional ingredients.
4. Sprinkle in the garlic and lemon juice, and then pour in the chicken stock.
5. Cover and cook on LOW for 8 hours.

Nutritional Information:
Calories 270, Total Fat 11 g, Saturated Fat 2 g, Total Carbohydrate 6 g, Dietary Fiber 1 g, Sugars 1 g, Protein 35 g

Jamaican Tenderloin

Cook Time: 6 hours
Serves: 6
SmartPoint™: 8

Ingredients:
1 ½ pounds pork tenderloin
2 tablespoons jerk seasoning
1 cup chicken stock
¼ cup low sodium soy sauce
¼ cup dark rum
1 tablespoon crushed red pepper flakes
1 cup mango, cubed
1 cup onion, sliced
1 cup green bell pepper, sliced
1 cup taro root, cubed
Cooked rice for serving (optional)

Directions:
1. Season the tenderloin liberally with the jerk seasoning and set it aside.
2. In a bowl, combine the chicken stock, soy sauce, rum, crushed red pepper, and mango. Mix well and pour into the bottom of the slow cooker.
3. Place the tenderloin on top of the sauce and the cover with the remaining vegetables: onion, green bell pepper, and taro root.
4. Cover and cook on LOW for 6 hours.
5. Serve with cooked rice, if desired.

Nutritional Information:

Calories 320.5, Total Fat 10.0 g, Saturated Fat 2.6 g, Total Carbohydrate 14.9 g, Dietary Fiber 2.1 g, Sugars 5.4 g, Protein 35.7 g

Italian Style Spareribs

Cook Time: 8 hours
Serves: 10
SmartPoint™: 8

Ingredients:
2 pounds extra lean pork spareribs
½ teaspoon salt
1 teaspoon black pepper
1 teaspoon dried oregano
4 cloves garlic, crushed and minced
3 cups Roma tomatoes, roasted and chopped
1 cup onion, sliced
1 cup beef stock
½ cup dry red wine
1 fresh rosemary sprig
4 cups fresh spinach, chopped

Directions:
1. Season the spareribs with the salt, black pepper, and oregano.
2. Top the spareribs with garlic and Roma tomatoes. Toss a little to ensure even coverage.
3. Layer the onion on top.
4. Combine the beef stock and dry red wine. Pour the mixture over the contents of the slow cooker and add the rosemary.
5. Cover and cook on LOW for 8 hours. After several hours of cooking remove the cover and gently stir the contents.
6. Fifteen minutes before serving, add the spinach and gently stir to moisten it in the broth. Cover the slow cooker and heat until the spinach is wilted.

Nutritional Information:
Calories 280, Total Fat 20 g, Saturated Fat 6 g, Total Carbohydrate 4 g, Dietary Fiber 1 g, Sugars 0 g, Protein 21 g

Beef and Lamb

Saucy Garden Steaks

Cook Time: 8 hours
Serves: 6
SmartPoint™: 5

Ingredients:
1 ½ pounds small beef steaks
½ teaspoon salt
1 teaspoon black pepper
1 teaspoon onion powder
1 tablespoon olive oil
1 cup pearl onions
2 cloves garlic, crushed and minced
2 cups portabella mushrooms, sliced thick
2 cups fresh green beans, trimmed
1 cup beef stock
¼ cup Worcestershire sauce
½ cup sugar free ketchup
1 teaspoon smoked paprika or ancho chili powder

Directions:
1. Season the steak with salt, black pepper, and onion powder.
2. Heat the olive oil in a skillet over medium-high heat.
3. Place the steaks in the skillet and sear until browned on both sides. Remove the steaks from the pan and transfer them to the slow cooker.
4. To the pan, add the pearl onions and sauté for 2-3 minutes.
5. Add the garlic and mushrooms. Sauté just until the mushrooms begin to become tender.

6. Add the green beans, beef stock, Worcestershire sauce, ketchup and paprika or chili powder. Mix well and bring to a low boil.
7. Remove the sauce from the heat and transfer to it the slow cooker, making sure the steak is evenly covered.
8. Cover the slow cooker and cook on LOW for 8 hours.
9. Serve with fresh salad, if desired.

Nutritional Information:
Calories 193, Total Fat 4 g, Saturated Fat 1 g, Total Carbohydrate 8 g, Dietary Fiber 2 g, Sugars 3 g, Protein 28 g

Brisket and Cabbage Dinner

Cook Time: 8 hours
Serves: 10
SmartPoint™: 7

Ingredients:
2 pounds beef brisket
1 tablespoon pickling spices (if spice packet is not included with brisket)
1 tablespoon black peppercorns
3 cups red potatoes, quartered
2 cups carrots, sliced thick
1 cup onion, sliced
1 small head cabbage, cut into 6-8 wedges
2 cups beef stock
1 tablespoon prepared horseradish
1 bay leaf

Directions:
1. Season the brisket with the pickling spices or spice packet and place it in the slow cooker.
2. Add the black peppercorns over and around the brisket.
3. Add the potatoes, carrots, onion, and cabbage over and around the brisket.
4. Combine the beef stock, horseradish, and bay leaf. Once combined, pour the liquid over the contents of the slow cooker.
5. Cover and cook on LOW for 8 hours.

Nutritional Information:
Calories 273, Total Fat 11 g, Saturated Fat 4 g, Total Carbohydrate 11 g, Dietary Fiber 2 g, Sugars 1 g, Protein 29 g

Gingery Asian Sloppy Joes

Cook Time: 6 hours
Serves: 8
SmartPoint™: 8

Ingredients:
1 ½ pounds lean ground beef
½ teaspoon salt
1 teaspoon black pepper
2 teaspoons crushed red pepper flakes
1 cup beef stock
¼ cup soy sauce
1 tablespoon sesame oil
1 tablespoon tomato paste
1 teaspoon honey
1 tablespoon fresh ginger, grated
2 cloves garlic, crushed and minced
½ cup thinly sliced cucumbers, for serving
¼ cup scallions, sliced for serving
Pickled ginger slices for serving (optional)
Weight Watchers® appropriate sandwich buns for serving

Directions:
1. Crumble the ground beef, place it in the slow cooker, and season it with the salt, black pepper, and crushed red pepper flakes.
2. In a bowl, combine the beef stock, soy sauce, sesame oil, tomato paste, honey, ginger, and garlic. Mix well.
3. Pour the sauce over the ground beef and mix gently to ensure even coverage.

4. Cover and cook on LOW for 6 hours.
5. Serve on sandwich buns garnished with cucumbers, scallions, and pickled ginger, if desired.

Nutritional Information:
Calories 257, Total Fat 19 g, Saturated Fat 7 g, Total Carbohydrate 3 g, Dietary Fiber 1 g, Sugars 2 g, Protein 16 g

Mushroomy Pot Roast

Cook Time: 8 ½ hours
Serves: 10
SmartPoint™: 7

Ingredients:
2 pounds pot roast
1 tablespoon olive oil
1 teaspoon salt
1 teaspoon black pepper
1 tablespoon fresh thyme
3 cloves garlic, crushed and minced
2 cups sweet yellow onion, sliced
2 cups sweet potatoes, cubed
3 cups cremini mushrooms, quartered
2 cups mini bella mushrooms, quartered
2 cups beef stock
½ cup dry red wine
1 bay leaf
1 fresh rosemary sprig

Directions:
1. Season the pot roast with olive oil, salt, black pepper, thyme, and garlic. Rub the seasoning well into all sides of the roast.
2. Heat a large cast iron skillet or Dutch oven medium heat.
3. Place the roast in the pan and brown each side. Transfer it to a slow cooker.
4. Add the onion and sweet potatoes to the skillet. Sauté for 2 minutes.
5. Add the mushrooms and cook just until they begin to become tender.

6. Add the beef stock, red wine, bay leaf, and rosemary. Bring the liquid to a low boil and cook for 2-3 minutes until the sauce is slightly reduced.
7. Remove the sauce and vegetables from the stove and pour them over the roast.
8. Cover and cook on LOW for 8 hours.

Nutritional Information:
Calories 320, Total Fat 19 g, Saturated Fat 1 g, Total Carbohydrate 11 g, Dietary Fiber 1 g, Sugars 1 g, Protein 28 g

Tri Tip Fajitas

Cook Time: 8 hours
Serves: 8
SmartPoint™: 7

Ingredients:
1 ½ pounds tri tip roast
1 tablespoon brown sugar
2 tablespoons paprika
1 tablespoons smoked chili powder
2 teaspoons onion powder
½ teaspoon coriander
1 teaspoon celery seed
½ teaspoon salt
1 teaspoon white pepper
1 tablespoon olive oil
1 cup red bell pepper, sliced
1 cup green bell pepper, sliced
1 cup onion, sliced
2 cups mushrooms, sliced
1 cup tomato juice
½ cup beef stock
1 cup tomatoes, diced
1 cup avocado, chopped (optional)
1 cup lettuce, sliced
½ cup fresh cilantro, chopped
Low fat flour tortillas for serving (optional)

Directions:

1. In a bowl, combine the brown sugar, paprika, smoked chili powder, onion powder, coriander, celery seed, salt, and white pepper. Mix well.
2. Pat the spice mixture evenly into the roast.
3. Heat the olive oil in a skillet over medium heat.
4. Add the roast and brown evenly on all sides. Remove it from the heat and set it aside.
5. Add the red bell pepper, green bell pepper, onion, and mushrooms to the slow cooker.
6. Place the meat on top of the vegetables, and then add the tomato juice and beef stock.
7. Cover and cook on LOW for 8 hours.
8. Serve in low fat tortillas, garnished with tomato, avocado, lettuce, and cilantro.

Nutritional Information:

Calories 301, Total Fat 18 g, Saturated Fat 1 g, Total Carbohydrate 8 g, Dietary Fiber 1 g, Sugars 3 g, Protein 25 g

Dark Cherry Beef Roast

Cook Time: 8 hours
Serves: 10
SmartPoint™: 7

Ingredients:
2 pounds boneless beef roast
1 teaspoon salt
1 teaspoon black pepper
1 tablespoon olive oil
2 cups carrots, sliced
3 cups Brussels sprouts, quartered
¼ cup shallots, diced
1 cup dark cherries, pitted and halved
½ cup sugar free cranberry juice
½ cup balsamic vinegar
1 cup beef stock
2 bay leaves
1 tablespoon fresh thyme

Directions:
1. Heat the olive oil in a skillet over medium heat.
2. Season the roast with salt and black pepper. Place the roast in the skillet and brown evenly on all sides. Place the roast in the slow cooker.
3. Cover and surround the roast with carrots, Brussels sprouts, shallots and cherries.
4. Combine the cranberry juice, balsamic vinegar, and beef stock. Mix well and pour the liquid into the slow cooker.
5. Add the bay leaves and fresh thyme.
6. Cover and cook on LOW for 8 hours.

Nutritional Information:
Calories 310, Total Fat 19 g, Saturated Fat 1 g, Total Carbohydrate 8 g, Dietary Fiber 2 g, Sugars 3 g, Protein 27 g

Curried Lamb

Cook Time: 6 hours
Serves: 8
SmartPoint™: 6

Ingredients:
2 pounds lamb shoulder meat, cubed
½ teaspoon salt
1 teaspoon black pepper
1 tablespoon coconut oil
1 cup onion, sliced
1 cup apple, chopped
2 cloves garlic, crushed and minced
2 tablespoons freshly grated ginger
2 tablespoons curry powder
2 teaspoons crushed red pepper flakes
2 cups sweet potatoes, peeled and cubed
1 cup tomatoes, chopped
2 cups chicken stock
1 cup coconut milk
3 cups fresh spinach
Cooked rice for serving (optional)
Fresh mint, chopped for garnish (optional)

Directions:
1. Season the lamb with salt and black pepper.
2. Heat the coconut oil in a skillet over medium heat. Add the meat and cook until browned evenly on all sides. Remove it from the stovetop and transfer it to a slow cooker.

3. Return the pan to the heat and add more coconut oil if necessary. Continue heating over medium and add the onion and apple. Sauté for 2-3 minutes.
4. Add the garlic, ginger, curry powder, and crushed red pepper flakes. Cook for an additional 1-2 minutes, or until highly fragrant.
5. Add the contents of the skillet, along with the sweet potatoes and tomatoes, to the slow cooker.
6. Combine the coconut milk and chicken stock. Mix well and add to the slow cooker.
7. Cover and cook on LOW for 6 hours.
8. Twenty minutes before serving, remove the cover and stir in the spinach.
9. Serve over rice, if desired, and garnish with fresh mint.

Nutritional Information:
Calories 250, Total Fat 9 g, Saturated Fat 4 g, Total Carbohydrate 15 g, Dietary Fiber 2 g, Sugars 2 g, Protein 25 g

Eggplant and Lamb

Cook Time: 6 hours
Serves: 8
SmartPoint™: 6

Ingredients:
2 pounds lamb shoulder meat, cubed
1 teaspoon salt
1 teaspoon black pepper
1 tablespoon olive oil
2 cups eggplant, peeled and cubed
1 cup onion, sliced
1 cup artichoke hearts, quartered
1 cup Roma tomatoes, chopped
4 cloves garlic, crushed and minced
1 teaspoon dried oregano
1 teaspoon dried thyme
1 cup pure tomato juice
½ cup beef stock
¼ cup dry white wine (optional)
3 cups cooked quinoa, for serving

Directions:
1. Season the lamb with salt and black pepper.
2. Place the olive oil in a skillet and heat it over medium.
3. Add the lamb and cook until browned on all sides. Remove the meat from the pan and transfer it to the slow cooker.
4. Return the pan to the stovetop and add the eggplant and onion. Sauté for 3-4 minutes. Remove from the heat and transfer the vegetables to the slow cooker.

5. To the slow cooker, add the artichoke hearts, tomato, garlic, oregano, and thyme.
6. Combine the tomato juice, beef stock, and white wine. Pour the liquid over the contents of the slow cooker.
7. Cover and cook on LOW for 6 hours.
8. Serve with cooked quinoa.

Nutritional Information:
Calories 254, Total Fat 9 g, Saturated Fat 2 g, Total Carbohydrate 19 g, Dietary Fiber 3 g, Sugars 2 g, Protein 26 g

Dijon Brisket

Cook Time: 8 hours
Serves: 6
SmartPoint™: 7

Ingredients:
1 ½ pounds beef brisket
½ teaspoon salt
1 teaspoon coarsely ground black pepper
¼ cup Dijon mustard
1 tablespoon prepared horseradish
4 cups asparagus, trimmed
2 cups purple fingerling potatoes, sliced thick
2 teaspoons lemon juice
½ cup beef stock

Directions:
1. Season the brisket with salt and black pepper.
2. Using a brush or your fingertips, rub in the Dijon mustard and horseradish. Set aside.
3. Arrange the asparagus and fingerling potatoes in the bottom of the slow cooker. Drizzle with the lemon juice and add the beef stock.
4. Place the brisket in the slow cooker and cover.
5. Cook on LOW for 6 hours.

Nutritional Information:
Calories 311, Total Fat 14 g, Saturated Fat 5 g, Total Carbohydrate 12 g, Dietary Fiber 3 g, Sugars 1 g, Protein 37 g

Vegetarian

Quinoa Casserole with Mushrooms and Artichokes

Cook Time: 4 hours
Serves: 8
SmartPoint™: 6

Ingredients:
1 tablespoon olive oil
1 cup red onion, chopped
2 cloves garlic, crushed and minced
3 cups wild mushroom mix, sliced
1 tablespoon flour
¼ cup dry white wine
2 cups skim milk
½ teaspoon nutmeg
1 teaspoon ground sage
2 cups vegetable stock
1 cup artichoke hearts, quartered
½ cup walnuts, finely chopped
¼ cup capers
4 cups cooked quinoa
½ cup freshly grated Parmesan cheese

Directions:
1. Heat the olive oil in a skillet over medium heat.
2. Add the onion and garlic. Sauté the mixture for 3-4 minutes.
3. Add the mushrooms and sauté an additional 2-3 minutes, or just until the mushrooms become tender.
4. Sprinkle the mixture with flour and stir gently.

5. Slowly, add the wine and skim milk in increments, stirring after each addition, until a sauce begins to form and thicken.
6. Season with nutmeg and sage before adding in the vegetable stock. Bring the sauce to a low boil while stirring and then remove from the heat.
7. Add the artichoke hearts, walnuts, capers, quinoa, and Parmesan cheese to the slow cooker. Toss to mix.
8. Next, add the sauce from the pan. Stir to ensure even distribution.
9. Cover and cook on LOW for 4 hours.

Nutritional Information:
Calories 214, Total Fat 9 g, Saturated Fat 1 g, Total Carbohydrate 25 g, Dietary Fiber 3 g, Sugars 4 g, Protein 8 g

Ratatouille

Cook Time: 4 hours
Serves: 6
SmartPoint™: 4

Ingredients:
3 cups eggplant, peeled and cubed
2 cups zucchini, sliced
2 cups summer squash, sliced
1 tablespoon olive oil
1 cup onion, sliced
2 cloves garlic, crushed and minced
1 cup green bell pepper, sliced
2 cups roasted, crushed tomatoes, with liquid
1 tablespoon herbs de Provence
½ cup tomato juice
½ cup vegetable stock
¼ cup dry red wine
1 teaspoon salt
1 teaspoon black pepper

Directions:
1. Combine the eggplant, zucchini, and summer squash together and place them in the slow cooker.
2. Warm the olive oil in a large skillet over medium heat.
3. Add the onions, garlic, and green bell pepper. Sauté for 3-4 minutes.
4. Add the crushed roasted tomatoes, herbs de Provence, tomato juice, vegetable stock, and dry red wine to the skillet. Bring to a low boil, before reducing the heat and simmering for 3-4 minutes.

5. Remove the skillet from the heat and transfer the contents to the slow cooker.
6. Season with salt and black pepper.
7. Cover the slow cooker and cook on HIGH for 4 hours.

Nutritional Information:
Calories 86, Total Fat 0 g, Saturated Fat 0 g, Total Carbohydrate \13 g, Dietary Fiber 3 g, Sugars 3 g, Protein 2 g

Colorful Vegetable Risotto

Cook Time: 4 hours
Serves: 4
SmartPoint™: 5

Ingredients:
1 tablespoon olive oil
¼ cup shallots, diced
2 cloves garlic, crushed and minced
1 cup short grain brown rice
¼ cup dry white wine
2 cups vegetable stock
½ cup carrots, shredded
½ cup zucchini, shredded (excess liquid removed)
½ cup yellow bell pepper, diced
½ teaspoon salt
1 teaspoon black pepper
2 teaspoons fresh tarragon
1 cup various colored grape tomatoes, quartered
½ cup fresh peas
1 tablespoon fresh chives
¼ cup fresh parsley
¼ cup shredded Asiago cheese

Directions:
1. Heat the olive oil in a skillet over medium heat.
2. Add the shallots and garlic. Sauté until translucent, approximately 3-5 minutes.
3. Add the brown rice and cook, stirring frequently for 2-3 minutes, or until lightly toasted.
4. Add the wine and cook, while stirring, until the wine has evaporated.

5. Remove the pan from the heat and transfer the rice mixture to a slow cooker.
6. To the slow cooker, add the carrots, zucchini, and bell pepper. Season the vegetables and rice with salt, black pepper, and tarragon. Mix well.
7. Add the vegetable stock and stir.
8. Cover and cook on HIGH for 2 ½ hours.
9. Remove the lid and stir in the tomatoes, peas, chives, parsley and Asiago cheese.
10. Cover and cook an additional 20 minutes before serving.

Nutritional Information:
Calories 138, Total Fat 4 g, Saturated Fat 1 g, Total Carbohydrate 20 g, Dietary Fiber 3 g, Sugars 3 g, Protein 3 g

Basil Angel Hair Frittata

Cook Time: 2 hours
Serves: 6
SmartPoint™: 3

Ingredients:
2 cups beaten eggs, or egg substitute
½ teaspoon salt
1 teaspoon black pepper
2 cups whole wheat angel hair pasta, cooked
1 cup Roma tomatoes, sliced
2 cloves garlic, crushed and minced
2 cups fresh spinach, torn
½ cup fresh basil, torn
½ cup fresh grated Parmesan cheese
Cooking spray

Directions:
1. Lightly coat the inside of a slow cooker with vegetable spray.
2. Season the beaten egg mixture with salt and black pepper. Layer in the whole wheat angel hair pasta, tomatoes, garlic, spinach, basil, and Parmesan cheese in the slow cooker.
3. Pour the egg mixture over and gently stir the ingredients to make sure that the egg mixture goes all the way through to the bottom.
4. Cover the slow cooker and cook on HIGH for 2 hours.
5. Loosen the edges gently with a spatula before cutting and serving.

Nutritional Information:

Calories 142, Total Fat 2 g, Saturated Fat 1 g, Total Carbohydrate 17 g, Dietary Fiber 2 g, Sugars 1 g, Protein 13 g

Chayote and Quinoa Stuffed Peppers

Cook Time: 6 hours
Serves: 4
SmartPoint™: 5

Ingredients:
4 large green bell peppers
1 tablespoon olive oil
¼ cup shallots
2 cloves garlic, crushed and minced
½ cup chayote, chopped
½ cup tomatillo, chopped
4 cups cooked quinoa
½ teaspoon salt
1 teaspoon white pepper
½ teaspoon cumin
½ teaspoon smoked paprika
½ cup fresh cilantro, chopped
1 cup onion, sliced
1 cup fresh or jarred salsa verde
½ cup vegetable stock

Directions:
1. Remove the tops of the peppers and scoop out the seeds from each.
2. Heat the olive oil in a skillet over medium.
3. Add the shallots, garlic, and chayote to the skillet. Sauté for 3-4 minutes.
4. Add the tomatillos and cook an additional 3 minutes.
5. Turn off the heat and add the quinoa to the pan.
6. Season with salt, white pepper, cumin, smoked paprika, and cilantro. Mix well.

7. Spoon the quinoa mixture evenly into each of the peppers before placing them into the slow cooker.
8. In a blender, combine the onions, salsa verde and vegetable stock.
9. Pour the sauce over and around the peppers.
10. Cover and cook on LOW for 6 hours, or until the peppers are tender.

Nutritional Information:
Calories 188, Total Fat 4 g, Saturated Fat 0 g, Total Carbohydrate 32 g, Dietary Fiber 5 g, Sugars 4 g, Protein 5 g

Chickpea Chili

Cook Time: 6 hours
Serves: 8
SmartPoint™: 4

Ingredients:
4 cups roasted crushed tomatoes, chopped, with liquid
1 cup vegetable juice
¼ cup chipotle peppers in adobo sauce, chopped
1 cup carrots, chopped
1 cup celery, chopped
1 cup fresh corn kernels
½ cup green bell pepper
½ cup red onion
4 cloves garlic, crushed and minced
3 cups chickpeas, cooked or canned, drained
2 tablespoons chili powder
1 tablespoon cumin
1 teaspoon cayenne powder
1 teaspoon salt
1 teaspoon black pepper
3 cups vegetable stock
Avocado, sliced for garnish (optional)

Directions:
1. Combine the crushed tomatoes, vegetable juice, and chipotle peppers. Mix well.
2. Pour the mixture into a slow cooker.
3. Next, layer in the carrots, celery, corn, green bell pepper, red onion, garlic, and chickpeas.
4. Season with chili powder, cumin, cayenne powder, salt, and black pepper. Mix well.

5. Pour in the vegetable stock, adding more if desired for a thinner chili.
6. Cover the slow cooker and cook on LOW for 6 hours.
7. Garnish with sliced avocado before serving, if desired.

Nutritional Information:
Calories 162, Total Fat 1 g, Saturated Fat 0 g, Total Carbohydrate 35 g, Dietary Fiber 6 g, Sugars 5 g, Protein 7 g

Veggie Fajita Salad

Cook Time: 2 hours
Serves: 6
SmartPoint™: 4

Ingredients:

1 cup red bell pepper, sliced
1 cup yellow bell pepper, sliced
1 cup Poblano pepper, sliced
1 cup onion, sliced
2 cups multi-colored cherry tomatoes, halved
1 teaspoon smoked paprika
1 teaspoon chili powder
½ teaspoon cayenne
½ teaspoon coriander
1 teaspoon salt
1 teaspoon coarse ground black pepper
1 tablespoon lime juice
½ cup spicy vegetable juice
4 cups dark salad greens
1 avocado, sliced
1 cup fresh pineapple chunks
½ cup fresh cilantro, chopped
½ cup queso fresco cheese, shredded

Directions:

1. Combine the red bell pepper, yellow bell pepper, Poblano pepper, onion and cherry tomatoes in a slow cooker.
2. Season the vegetables with the smoked paprika, chili powder, cayenne, coriander, salt, black pepper, and lime juice. Mix well.

3. Add the vegetable juice, cover the slow cooker and cook on HIGH for 2 hours.
4. Place the salad greens on serving plates, topped with avocado.
5. Next, add the fajita vegetables along with fresh pineapple, cilantro, and queso fresco cheese.

Nutritional Information:
Calories 116, Total Fat 5 g, Saturated Fat 1 g, Total Carbohydrate 14 g, Dietary Fiber 4 g, Sugars 4 g, Protein 3 g

Vegetable Gumbo

Cook Time: 4 hours
Serves: 8
SmartPoint™: 6

Ingredients:
1 tablespoon olive oil
1 cup onion, chopped
1 cup green bell pepper, chopped
½ cup celery, chopped
4 cloves garlic, crushed and minced
2 tablespoons flour
2 ½ cups vegetable stock
2 cups tomatoes, chopped
1 cup kidney beans, cooked and rinsed
1 cup black beans, cooked and rinsed
1 cup fresh corn kernels
2 cups mushrooms, sliced
1 cup carrots, diced
1 cup frozen okra, sliced
2 tablespoons Cajun seasoning
1 tablespoon cayenne pepper sauce
1 bay leaf
1 teaspoon salt
1 teaspoon black pepper
4 cups cooked brown rice, for serving

Directions:
1. Heat the olive oil in a skillet over medium heat.
2. Add the onion, bell pepper, celery and garlic. Sauté for 3-5 minutes.
3. Sprinkle in the flour and toss to mix.

4. Slowly add the vegetable stock, stirring constantly.
5. Bring the liquid to a low boil, stirring constantly, until the liquid begins to thicken.
6. Remove the pan from the heat and transfer the contents to the slow cooker.
7. Add the tomatoes, kidney beans, black beans, corn, mushrooms, carrots, and okra.
8. Season with the Cajun seasoning, cayenne pepper sauce, bay leaf, salt, and black pepper.
9. Cover and cook on HIGH for 4 hours.
10. Serve over cooked rice.

Nutritional Information:
Calories 201, Total Fat 3 g, Saturated Fat 0 g, Total Carbohydrate 45 g, Dietary Fiber 8 g, Sugars 2 g, Protein 8 g

Greek Succotash

Cook Time: 4 ½ hours
Serves: 8
SmartPoint™: 6

Ingredients:
1 cup red bell pepper, chopped
1 cup zucchini, chopped
1 cup eggplant, peeled and cubed
2 cups roasted tomatoes, chopped with any liquid
1 cup onion, chopped
4 cloves garlic, crushed and minced
½ cup large Kalamata olives, quartered
2 cups white beans, cooked or canned and rinsed
1 teaspoon salt
1 teaspoon black pepper
½ teaspoon nutmeg
½ teaspoon oregano
½ cup fresh parsley, chopped
¼ cup balsamic vinegar
¼ cup lemon juice
4 cups cooked bulgur
½ cup feta cheese, crumbled

Directions:
1. Combine the red bell pepper, zucchini, eggplant, tomatoes, onion, garlic, olives, and beans together in a slow cooker.
2. Season with salt, black pepper, nutmeg, and oregano. Mix well.
3. Cover the slow cooker and cook on LOW for 4 hours.

4. Remove the lid and stir in the parsley, balsamic vinegar, lemon juice, and bulgur. Cover and cook an additional 20 minutes.
5. Garnish with feta cheese before serving.

Nutritional Information:
Calories 220.8, Total Fat 4.1 g, Saturated Fat 1.2 g, Total Carbohydrate 39.2 g, Dietary Fiber 8.9 g, Sugars 0.9 g, Protein 9.5 g

Conclusion

As you work your way through the many delicious and healthy recipes in this book, you will find that your slow cooker is more versatile and diet friendly than you ever imagined. Gone forever will be the idea that slow cookers are only for heavy stews and fat laden casseroles. In a time when it seems everyone is so busy, there is no reason to let our health suffer as a consequence of our overburdened schedules. You can relax at the end of the day, knowing that in your kitchen awaits a flavorful, home cooked meal that satisfies your appetite, your SmartPoint™ limit, and most importantly, your soul.

Keep in mind as you use the recipes in this book, that they were designed to carry you through not only the achievement of your weight loss goals, but also your healthy maintenance. Nothing about these recipes screams low calorie or sacrifice. Once you have reached your health goals, you will not look back on these recipes with the distain that is often bestowed upon "diet foods", but rather the anticipation of deliciousness for years to come.

More Books from Madison Miller

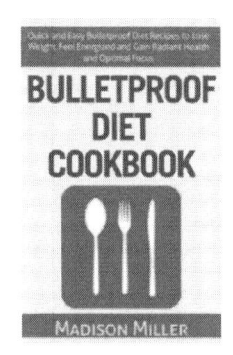

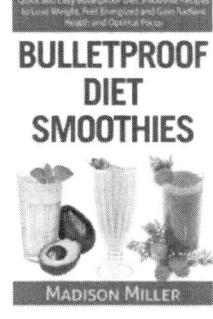

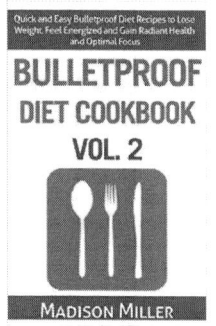

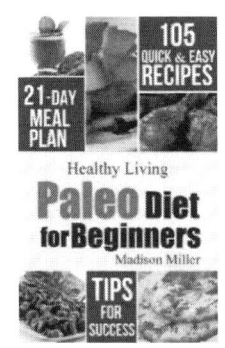

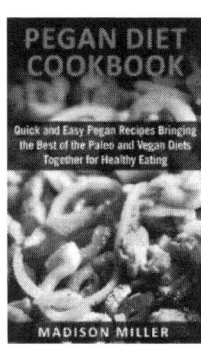

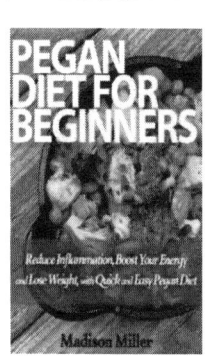

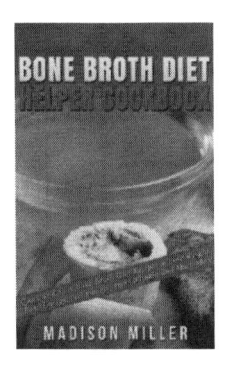

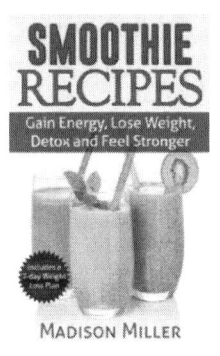

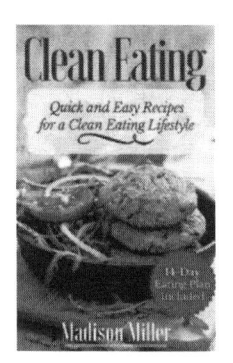

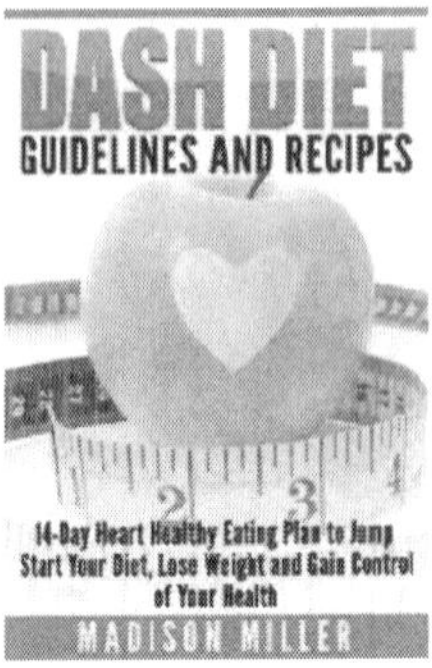
DASH DIET
GUIDELINES AND RECIPES
14-Day Heart Healthy Eating Plan to Jump Start Your Diet, Lose Weight and Gain Control of Your Health
MADISON MILLER

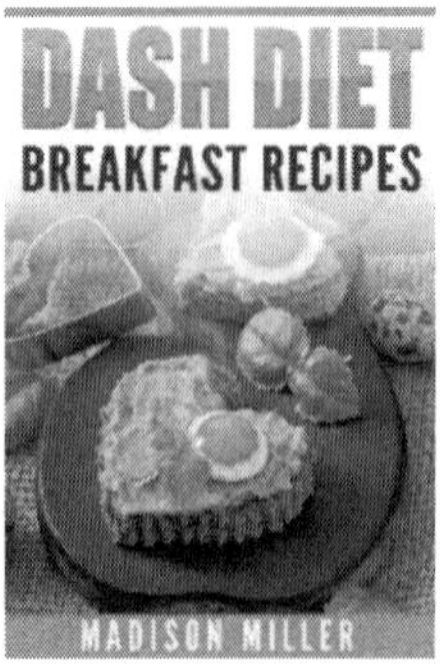
DASH DIET
BREAKFAST RECIPES
MADISON MILLER

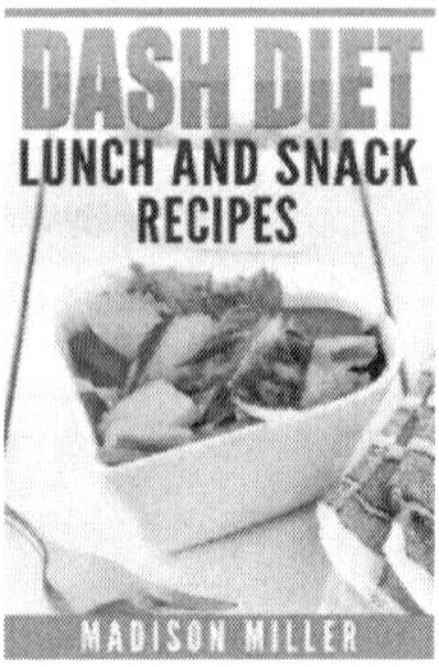
DASH DIET
LUNCH AND SNACK RECIPES
MADISON MILLER

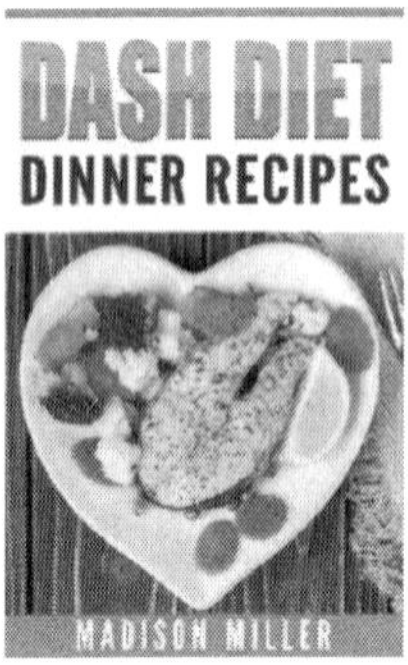
DASH DIET
DINNER RECIPES
MADISON MILLER

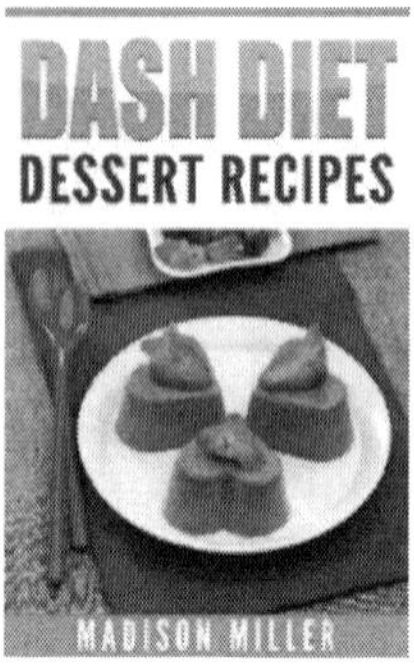
DASH DIET
DESSERT RECIPES
MADISON MILLER

Appendix – Cooking Conversion Charts

1. Measuring Equivalent Chart

Type	Imperial	Imperial	Metric
Weight	1 dry ounce		28g
	1 pound	16 dry ounces	0.45 kg
Volume	1 teaspoon		5 ml
	1 dessert spoon	2 teaspoons	10 ml
	1 tablespoon	3 teaspoons	15 ml
	1 Australian tablespoon	4 teaspoons	20 ml
	1 fluid ounce	2 tablespoons	30 ml
	1 cup	16 tablespoons	240 ml
	1 cup	8 fluid ounces	240 ml
	1 pint	2 cups	470 ml
	1 quart	2 pints	0.95 l
	1 gallon	4 quarts	3.8 l
Length	1 inch		2.54 cm

* Numbers are rounded to the closest equivalent

2. Oven Temperature Equivalent Chart

T(°F)	T(°C)
220	100
225	110
250	120
275	140
300	150
325	160
350	180
375	190
400	200
425	220
450	230
475	250
500	260

*   T(°C) = [T(°F)-32] * 5/9

**   T(°F) = T(°C) * 9/5 + 32

*** Numbers are rounded to the closest equivalent

Printed in Germany
by Amazon Distribution
GmbH, Leipzig